T0199067

healthy
rules of the
road

Family Edition

Wendy Cooper

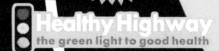

Healthy Highway
the green light to good health

Balboa Press books may be ordered through booksellers or by contacting:

Balboa Press
A Division of Hay House
1663 Liberty Drive
Bloomington, IN 47403
www.balboapress.com
1 (877) 407-4847

ISBN: 978-1-5043-9110-8 (sc)
ISBN: 978-1-5043-9111-5 (e)

Library of Congress Control Number: 2017917649

Print information available on the last page.

Balboa Press rev. date: 03/12/2019

This book is designed as a guide only to motivate families to become aware of healthy choices that they make. It is not to diagnose or treat any condition. Please seek professional advice from your medical practitioner for such occurrences.

BALBOA.
PRESS
A DIVISION OF HAY HOUSE

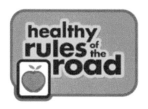

Healthy Highway Road Map

TABLE OF CONTENTS

Introduction

About Wendy Cooper, Founder..*2*

About Healthy Highway...*2*

Dedication..*3*

Letter from Wendy Cooper..*4*

Incorporating traffic concepts

Red Light/Green Light Concept..*5*

Traffic Vocabulary..*6*

Nutrition Rules of the Road...*7*

Start Your Engines..*8*

Daily Activities...*10*

In the Driver's Seat

Message from Rev, the Healthy Highway Dog...*11*

Traffic School

Cool Fuels..*12*

Safety Rules of the Kitchen..*13*

Your kitchen is the showroom..*14*

Lunch Box Ideas...*16*

Lunch Box Rules...*17*

Coop's Creations:..*18*

Green Light Decisions

Honest Street..*19*

Cooperate Circle...*20*

Family Road Map Calendars

List of Activities and Ideas..*21*

Finish Line
Goal Setting 24

Healthy Highway License Plate Award
Celebrate Your Accomplishments 25

Road to Success
Commit to Your Choices 26

My Story
From the heart 27

Rev's Activity Kit for Kids
Fun activities 28

Are you looking for a healthier lifestyle for your family?

JOIN THE HEALTHY REVOLUTION...

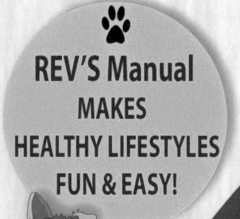

REV'S Manual
MAKES
HEALTHY LIFESTYLES
FUN & EASY!

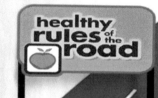

healthy rules of the road

"I promise to make one HEALTHY CHOICE everyday"

The award-winning Healthy Highway program was designed by Wendy Cooper, 30-year physical education teacher and mother of two. She provides a road map for busy families on the go, looking for a fun and easy system to implement a healthy lifestyle for every member of the house.

www.healthy-highway.com

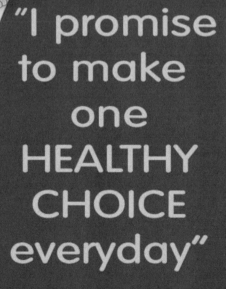

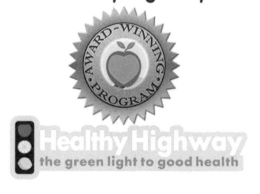

AWARD-WINNING PROGRAM

Healthy Highway
the green light to good health

About Healthy Highway

After working with the *Healthy Rules of the Road* program in schools for over 10 years, I knew my next road was to go directly to families. Our bodies are complex but to simplify it by comparing them to a car engine makes it easy and fun. Foods are fuels, we want to be at top performance, and we want to run at top speed. We all have an inner "GPS", or natural instinct, that we simply have to listen to. Our bodies will tell us what fuels we need and which ones will be the most beneficial.

I'll provide you with an easy-to-follow action plan of monthly activities, fun recipes, traffic-themed visuals, and ways to engage your family in educational conversations that lead to green light choices.

Here is your Healthy Highway Warranty:

1. Read and understand the information in this manual.
2. Practice the concepts by applying them to your daily decisions.
3. Watch healthy choices increase. This is a lifetime warranty!

Life is a highway of learning.... get ready to *accelerate* down the *Healthy Highway* to a healthy lifestyle.

About Wendy Cooper, President & Founder of Healthy Highway

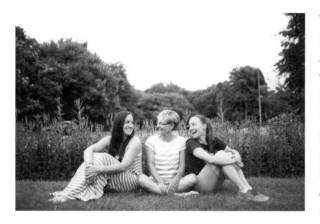

Wendy Cooper, 30 year physical education teacher and mother of two, is the founder and president of the award-winning, fun Healthy Highway program that uses traffic themes and metaphors to encourage children to make healthy choices. Healthy Highway has been used in schools around the country and featured in numerous publications. In March 2012, Healthy Highway received national recognition and was featured as a "How Cool is That?" organization on Rachael Ray's Yum-O website and in the Yum-O Newsletter. Wendy has also been the recipient of a number of accolades and awards.

Throughout her career Wendy's goal has always been to help children and families understand that it can be fun to make healthy choices and to ensure healthy lifestyles and nutrition for all children – Healthy Highway is a testament to achieving that goal.

Wendy, now for the first time, will offer her program directly to individual families with a brand new website and a home version of the Healthy Highway Kit. The new Riding with Rev Family Pack, as described on page 24, is tailored for busy parents and their children looking for a program that encourages a healthy lifestyle for the entire family.

Wendy Cooper resides in a suburb of Rochester, NY. She enjoys bike riding, hiking, traveling and spending time with her two daughters, Brittany and Brianna.

Dedication...

The all new Healthy Rules of the Road Family Edition is dedicated to my sister Debbie. Her positive green-light thinking has brought her through an incredible health crisis. Her strength and determination have been a true inspiration.

Dear Families,

I am so glad you are starting down the highway to healthy choices. Your *owner's manual* was designed as a guide with one purpose: for you to make the best choices to meet <u>your</u> family's needs.

EACH MONTH HAS A FOCUS

First Month   Introduce the concepts of "Rules of the Road." Use the *30 Ways for 30 Healthy Days* Calendar for this month.

Second Month   Make heart healthy choices by choosing as many green light foods as possible as *fuels.*

Third Month   Activity month has the goal of *revving* your engines with many different activities.

Congratulations: Celebrate your successes with fun family activities!

You will be provided with a calendar (which you may print out for each month) to help track your healthy choices. Your final "destination" will be to complete 3 of these calendars.

This is meant as a guide only, a *road map* if you will. Only you can decide where it will lead you. There will be detours, road blocks and U-turns, but as long as you keep moving forward you will achieve the goal of a healthy, well-tuned, high performance *engine*.

You will find this program is different as it designates YOU as the main driver. I will provide the concepts to work with and incorporate into your daily routine, but you have the "title" to this vehicle. You will make the decisions that are specifically designed for your body to reach its top performance. Listen to what I call your "inner GPS" which is a powerful navigation tool that will guide you to the best choices for you. Healthy Rules of the Road is a visual and vocabulary based program since 80% of our learning is visual. The green light concept of making decisions is a new way of thinking and can be applied to healthy choices in all areas of your life.

As parents, we have the unique opportunity to help our children achieve healthy lifestyles. We can serve as what I like to call "road models" by applying the concepts found in this manual. Each family is stronger when everyone participates and becomes involved in the choices. Our nutritional choices or *fuels* are the most important decisions we make. So, pull up a chair, create your own *learning lab* in your kitchen and, as a family, design your own *road trip* to healthy choices. I would enjoy hearing about all the trips you take as you continue to drive the many roads to a healthy lifestyle.

I am excited for you to begin. Thank you for allowing me to go on this journey with you. Remember to sign up for the Healthy Highway newsletter for more ideas and information at www.Healthy-Highway.com.

Sincerely,
Wendy Cooper
Wendy Cooper President & Founder
<u>www.healthy-highway.com</u>
<u>wcooper@healthy-highway.com</u>

Incorporating traffic concepts into your daily conversations

Using traffic vocabulary makes it easy and fun to engage your children in discussions about their choices. Thinking of your body as an engine allows each person to take ownership of the decisions being made. The common vocabulary provides a foundation for everyone to talk the same "language." What traffic terms will your family create?

Traffic vocabulary: examples of traffic discussions:

- How is your engine running today?
- What is in your fuel tank?
- Is your battery running low?
- Are you running on an empty fuel tank?
- Is your water tank full?
- Is your timing off...engine is running too fast or too slow?

When you make the connection that your body is like a car engine, it is easy to check your engine and tune it to how it is performing. This concept is easy to understand since we know what our cars need...high performance fuels, water, and oil. Simple...we need the same.

Traffic visuals are a fun tool to engage your children in the traffic theme

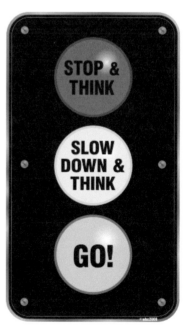

- Traffic signs on the road provide immediate reinforcement of the Rules of the Road. Each time you see a stop sign, say "Stop...always eat breakfast!"
- Traffic Light Foods: Green light choices make us feel better, look good and have energy. Good choices develop a sense of pride. There are no "good" or "bad" foods. Food is fuel and the choice we make will either have us running at top performance or clog our engine. If a red light choice is made, then a green light choice puts us back into alignment.
- Green Light Fuels: plant based; low sugar; low salt; low fat.
- Red Light Foods: high processed; high sugar; high salt; high fat.

Healthy Highway Testimonial:

"As a mom of three kids, I love that Healthy Highway tips apply to our whole family. My oldest loves how he can independently work towards a healthy goal (he tracks his Green Light Choices) and my younger kids LOVE Rev, Coop and Cruise. Such a fun way to work together in making awesome Green Light Choices. Thank you Healthy Highway!" Allison P., Rochester, NY

How to talk with your children about healthy decisions

The key is AWARENESS. Make the best choices possible. As you increase the intake of nutritious food choices, and you incorporate more movement into your day, your body will respond. You will begin to feel better, look better and have more energy. The power of thought plays an important role on this journey. As you feel better you become happier. You are the solution to having a "high performance engine."

"Green light" decision making is a new way of thinking. Ask yourself if your decision is a red, yellow or green light. When you are "stuck" on a decision, think of it in a traffic sense - is it a red light decision that is stopping you, are you frustrated, in a "traffic jam" where there is no forward movement? How can you change it to the yellow where you may have to use caution and slow down to gather more information? This gives you time to go at your own speed, shift gears, and think of more options. As soon as you realize what "light" choice you made, you have the ability to change it. Try this once a day and watch how it will "accelerate".

6 WAYS YOUR FAMILY CAN PRACTICE A HEALTHIER LIFESTYLE

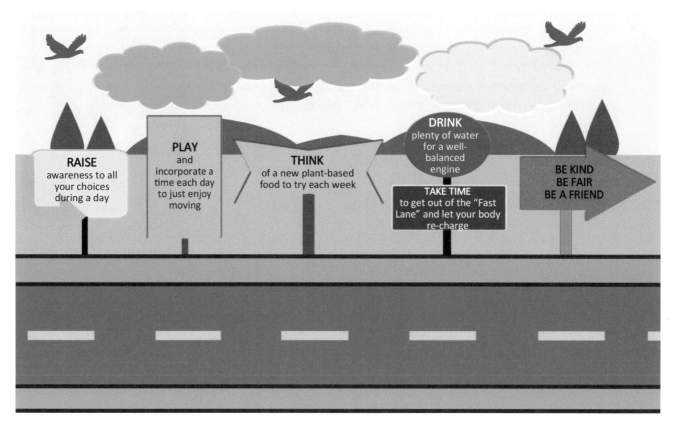

Nutrition Rules of the Road

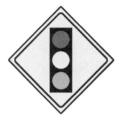

Rule #1: Stop for healthy snacks
Discussion topics: Have each family member list their favorite healthy snack; make a graph of each of the choices with the number of people liking each snack.

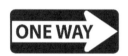

Rule #2: One way to 5 a day
Discussion topics: Why is it important to eat 5 fruits/veggies a day? Name 5 fruits and veggies. Draw your favorite fruit or veggie exercising!

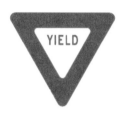

Rule #3: Watch out for oils, slow down on fat, pass by sugar Discussion topics: What can oils, fat, and sugar do to our engines? Will we run at top performance eating foods with high content of these ingredients? Read the label of foods you eat and look at the numbers of each of these categories.

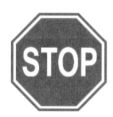

Rule #4: Stop, always eat breakfast
Discussion topics: Discuss the importance of breakfast and why it is considered the most important meal of the day. We are running on empty since we have not eaten since dinner. Name some high octane fuels for a healthy breakfast meal.

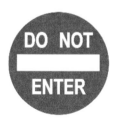

Rule #5: Do not enter with junk food, soda, or candy
Discussion topics: List the ingredients found in these foods. Name a healthier alternative food choice for each example.

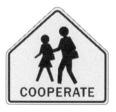

Rule #6: Be happy, be healthy, be strong
Discussion topics: Green light foods lead to strong muscles, feeling healthy, and lots of energy. See a list of green light foods on page 12. Name your favorite green light food.

Start Your Engines

How do you start on this road to healthy choices?

Begin to think of everything you eat as fuel. These choices will determine how your engine runs. Certain foods make us feel full, empty, lethargic, or revved up. Raise your awareness of what you are feeling after eating and make your choices based on that data.

Get your engine "road ready" with proper maintenance:

- Fill up with water for proper cooling
- Choose high performance fuels
- Check headlights (eye exams)
- Clean your air filter (breathe in fresh air)
- Scrub the grill (brush teeth)
- Make sure your inspection sticker is up to date (doctor check-up!)

Get a jump start by embracing these 2 concepts:

1. **Think of food as fuel and your body as an engine**

Our bodies absorb the nutrients they need. Try to choose as many "green light" foods as possible. Choose foods:
- with low amounts of sugar
- with low amounts of salt
- locally grown
- non GMO
- organic

2. **Embrace healthy lifestyle choices as your ignition key to good health**

Our bodies act like a "GPS" to lead us to healthy lifestyle choices. We need to "recalculate" when:
- we are running on empty and need more fuel
- we are tired and need restful sleep
- we are in low gear and need to exercise
- we are spinning our tires and need to relax
- we are going down a rocky road and need to be positive

Each food group is designed to benefit our engines as follows:

Carbohydrates/ Whole Grains:	**"Fuel pump"** - energy source that revs our engines *e.g. wild rice, quinoa*
Proteins:	**"Repair kit"** - builds muscles *e.g. beans and lentils, nuts, and seeds*
Oils/fats:	**"Lube job"** - keeps everything running smoothly *e.g. avocado, flax seed oil*
Fruits/Veggies:	**"Keys"** - Helps all nutrients work together to fight infection, provide energy, and keep the brain and nerves working well *e.g. tomato, watermelon/celery, broccoli*

***Road Map* to reading labels:**
think of a compass and use the
following "directions"

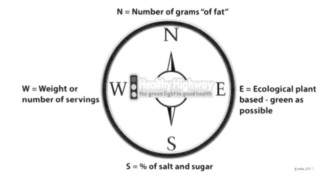

N = Number of grams "of fat"

W = Weight or number of servings

E = Ecological plant based - green as possible

S = % of salt and sugar

In the Driver's Seat

Incorporate fun activities into your daily routine!

- Establish a Healthy Highway "team" concept for your family. Encourage each family member to be part of the learning process: meal planning; shopping; prepping; listing activity choices; naming ideas to be a healthy home community.
- Define a ***destination*** or goal for your family. What improvements do you want to make to your food choices, activity choices, and family time choices? Involve everyone in this goal, and choose a goal for each month.
- ***Get in gear***! Take an action, big or small, doesn't matter what direction you choose. Each step will get you to your destination. You can't get lost, you have your **inner GPS** to guide you!
- Develop ***traffic theme*** vocabulary when discussing food choices, activities, or how you are feeling. Ex:
  I'm running on empty* or *I choose all green light foods.
- Visit the Healthy Highway website and sign up for the **Rules of the Road** newsletter for recipes, informational articles, and interactive features. **www.healthy-highway.com**
- Look up food facts and display them: i.e. the longest carrot ever grown was 193½ inches long!
  - ◊ Make graphs of family favorite foods and/or exercises
  - ◊ Chart job assignments for each family member to keep everyone running at top speed
- Let other families and your school communities know about your progress.
- Choose a family member to be a **Healthy Highway** *reporter*. With clipboard in hand, interview family members with the following questions: Why did you choose the foods you had today? What was the favorite food and why? Name the food group for each of the foods you ate at dinner. Share your results with the family.
- Establish the ***Food of the Week***. Choose one week a month to celebrate a favorite food group and list each of those foods that are included in the weekly meals.
- Make a mural by drawing pictures of foods exercising. Display on the refrigerator!
- Think of your grocery shopping as a ***road trip*** to find the healthiest *fuels,* new tastes, and new foods.
- Take the Healthy Highway Pledge: **"We promise to make at least ONE healthy choice every day!"**
- Take the Healthy Highway Oath: I (state your name) promise to uphold the laws of Healthy Highway. I promise to do my best to make healthy choices every day and to also help others to make healthy decisions.
- Take ***healthy -selfies*** anywhere and anytime your family is making healthy choices.
  Email them to: wcooper@healthy-highway.com

Hello!

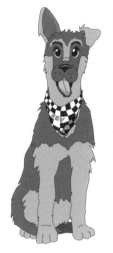

I'm Rev, the Healthy Highway mascot. I have been on the Healthy Highway for ten years with my owner, Wendy Cooper. She was a Physical Education teacher for 30 years and developed this program for her elementary students. She watched the children embrace the traffic-themed concepts and knew she had to share the success of the program with others. Schools across the country have implemented the school-wide edition of *Rules of the Road*. School cafeterias, pre-K programs, special needs organizations, after school programs, a local Special Olympics program, and a new local pilot program with the police department have all traveled down the Healthy Highway.

I am happy Wendy has decided to now bring the program directly to families. This owner's manual will help you incorporate the fun and educational concepts into your everyday habits. As you practice and apply the traffic concepts, pay attention to how your choices will gradually become "green light" healthy choices, which in turn will become a new "traffic pattern" for your family to follow.

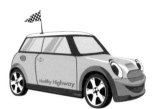

Just like Wendy, I love to teach and have great fun sharing my healthy choices with children. Please use my name when talking with your children about the choices they make. It makes it fun for them to know that I like certain foods, or I like to run, or I like to relax outside in the sunshine. I will also be introducing my friends "Coop" and Cruise". They travel with me and also enjoy sharing their favorite "green light" healthy choices.

My activity kit is where I talk to the children directly on how to be a "licensed driver" on the Healthy Highway. I will share my coloring pages, word searches, and a family "license plate" to color and hang on your refrigerator. I will also encourage them to help friends and other families take steps to increase healthy choices. I love to get emails so please have your children share any questions or ideas. I will always respond!

Enjoy the road trip!

Sincerely,
Rev

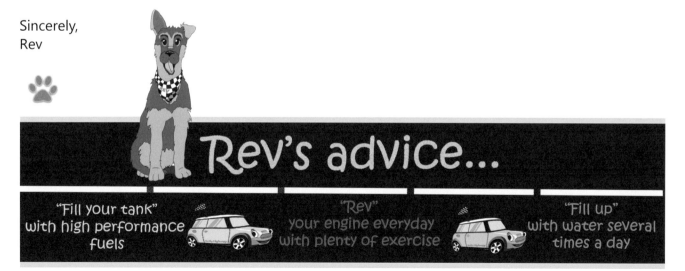

Cool Fuels

Here is an alphabetical list of healthy fuels to fill your tank and jump start your engine

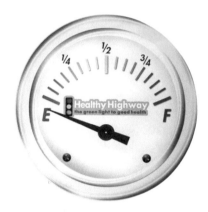

A	Asparagus, avocado	**N**	Nectarines, navy beans
B	Blueberries, broccoli	**O**	Oranges
C	Cauliflower, cucumber	**P**	Peppers, peas
D	Dates, dark chocolate	**Q**	Quiche, quinoa
E	Eggplant, endive	**R**	Raisins, raspberries
F	Fish, fruits	**S**	Salad, spinach
G	Grapes, green beans	**T**	Tomatoes, tangerine
H	Honey, hummus	**U**	Unsalted nuts
I	Instant rolled oats	**V**	Vegetables, vegetable soup
J	Jicama, natural jams	**W**	Water, watermelon
K	Kale, kiwi	**X**	X-tra veggies
L	Lima beans, lentils	**Y**	Yams, yellow peppers
M	Melons, mangos	**Z**	Zucchini, ziti

Safety Rules of the Kitchen

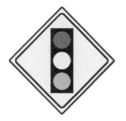

Rule #1 Go for healthy choices.
- Enjoy your favorite foods in moderation and use smart substitutes (healthy fats, natural sweeteners, organic).
- Add more spices, fruits and vegetables.

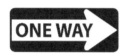

Rule #2 One way to keep foods safe.
- Store perishable foods in refrigerator or freezer.
- Maximum time out at room temperature is two hours. If temperatures are 85° or higher - 1 hour.
- ALWAYS thaw frozen foods overnight in refrigerator or in a cool water bath.

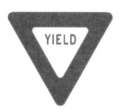

Rule #3 Watch out for hot surfaces. Respect all sharp kitchen tools.
- Always put dirty sharp knives next to sink since sudsy water may hide them.
- ALWAYS assume a burner is hot. Respect it accordingly.

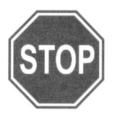

Rule #4 STOP - Always wash hands first.
- Germs are easily passed from people to food. Wash your hands after touching any object, especially other food.

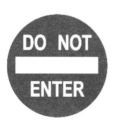

Rule #5 Do not enter without adult supervision.
- Have the adult turn on stoves, ovens and all equipment.
- Always have an adult with you when using a sharp utensil.

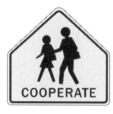

Rule #6 As a team, create your own "Kitchen Learning Lab".
- Be safe.
- Be creative.
- Have fun.

Your kitchen is the showroom

Think of your kitchen as a dealership *showroom* where you will be showing off the newest *models* of meals. Look at the colors of the foods you are using; discuss the *selling points* of the meals, *e.g. the nutritional value of the foods used, the taste; check to see if the ingredients are "fuel efficient"*, meaning they provide energy for your body (engine). At the end of the month have your family vote on the favorite recipe and start a recipe box of the *top of the line meals*. By the end of the year your *showroom* will be full of exciting model meals.

Get in gear: Different ways to cook food

Stove top: Place pot on burner to slowly heat through. Medium heat warms gently.

Grill: Heat food from below and food is close to the heat source. Heat grill before putting food on. Surface of food cooks quickly. Good for poultry, fish, veggies, and tender cuts of meat.

Sauté: Requires hot pan; heat pan for 1 minute, then add small amount of fat. Allow fat to get hot as well before adding food. Do not crowd pan. Toss or flip the food as you are cooking for even cooking.

Stir fry: Cut food into small pieces and cook over high heat. Stir often.

Steam: Moist heat cooking method. Food is separate from boiling water but in contact with steam.

Bake: Generally, speaks to cooking bread, pastry, and other bakery items.

Roast: Generally, speaks to cooking meats, poultry, and vegetable. Heat is hotter than baking so foods cook faster and brown easier.

Broil: Heat food from above. Heat broiler before adding food. Food is close to source of heat.

Inspection station: Suggested storage methods for fruits and vegetables

Refrigerate:
Apples, cantaloupe, honeydew, apricots
Asparagus, kale, lima beans, leafy vegetables, plums, spinach, sprouts, squash, zucchini, grapes, celery, beets Store unwashed in a plastic bag: broccoli, carrots, cauliflower, lettuce, peas
Store in a paper bag: mushrooms

Countertop:
Bananas, tomatoes, oranges, grapefruit, pineapple, lemons, limes eggplant, garlic, ginger, mangoes, peppers, cucumbers

Cool dry place:
All types of squash, sweet potatoes, potatoes, onions
Ripen on counter, then refrigerate: avocados, peaches, plums, pears, kiwi

Freshness tip:

Fruits and veggies give off a harmless, tasteless gas called ethylene after they are picked. All fruits and veggies produce this but some more than others. Keep these foods away from other fresh produce to slow down ripening and spoilage time.

Do not thaw or marinate foods on the counter. Bacteria can multiply rapidly at room temperature.

Lunch Box Ideas

An easy way to make lunch fun is to get a lunchbox with compartments. The large compartment can be your "base" as discussed above, and then add your "green light" choices in the smaller compartments. Here are some suggestions:

- Choose foods that will give you lots of "mileage" so you can be strong throughout your day.
- Use many colors.
- Be creative. Make it fun. Use mini cookie cutters to make shapes for cheese, meat, fruits, and veggies.
- Make faces or shapes when possible for added interest.
- Include each family member in packing lunches.
- Write notes of encouragement or gratitude to create smiles!

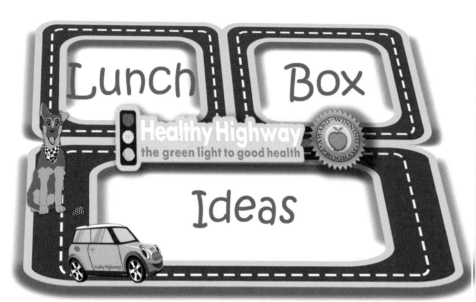

USE YOUR CREATIVITY & MAKE IT FUN!!!

Use mini cookie cutters to make shapes for cheese, meat, fruits and veggies when possible.

Use a lot of bright colors.

Make faces of shapes when possible for added interest. We eat with our eyes!!!!

Little notes of encouragement or gratitude found in lunchboxes also go a long way!!!

FOR THE MAIN ROAD
Meat and cheese bundles ▪ Pinwheel wraps on tortillas with meat and cheese ▪ Meat and cheese Mini kabobs ▪ Veggie skewers ▪ Fruit Kabobs ▪ Lettuce wraps filled with veggies or meat ▪ Spring rolls- thin veggies rolled in rice paper wraps ▪ Mini pizzas on pita ▪ Hearty salad topped with veggies ▪ Chex Caesar salad ▪ Taco salad with salsa and black beans ▪ Julienne salad ▪ Stuffed tomatoes with tuna or quinoa salad ▪ Quinoa salad

ON THE SIDE ROADS
Whole almonds ▪ Hummus ▪ Pita chips ▪ Cubed cheese ▪ Salsa ▪ Hardboiled egg ▪ A few olives ▪ Cucumber salad Cherry tomatoes ▪ Figs or dates ▪ Fresh baby carrots ▪ Celery sticks ▪ Apple wedges ▪ Fresh vegetable blend ▪ Fruit salad ▪ Fresh berries ▪ Yogurt ▪ Good granola ▪ Rice or lentil crackers ▪ Cashew or almond butter ▪ Organic applesauce ▪ Yogurt covered raisins ▪ Dried fruit ▪ Good trail mixes ▪ Dark chocolate pieces ▪ Whole grain pasta salad ▪ Couscous or quinoa salads ▪ Healthy muffins ▪ Tortilla chips

Lunch Box Rules

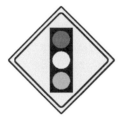

Rule #1 "Go" for a bright display of color, shapes and textures. Use mini cookie cutters to cut meats, cheese, fruits and veggies to create eye appealing lunch boxes. We eat with our eyes!
Change it up, utilize the seasons or holidays, and make it fresh and fun!

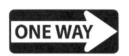

Rule #2 There is no "one way" in creating lunch boxes.
The more directions you go, the better it is. Roll meat in bundles, cut in cubes, or put on skewers. Place veggies in spring rolls, tortillas, or cut into pinwheel circles.

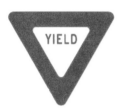

Rule #3 Slow down and think about healthy choices.
Watch for fruits that can be sliced, skewered, or cubed, for dessert, yogurt, or in breakfast bars. Pass by foods with high sugar content.

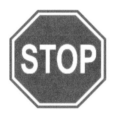

Rule #4 "Stop" putting boundaries of what your child "will eat".
Learn about and try new foods every week. Taste buds evolve every 6 months. Make "fuels" fun and positive and expand choices for their lunchbox.

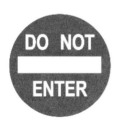

Rule #5 Avoid getting into a rut!
Compartment lunch boxes encourage more creativity. Kids will be excited to see what is in their lunch every day!

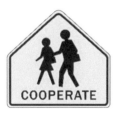

Rule #6 Work as a team – make the lunch together.
Listen to your child's feedback, and build on the foods they like. Add a note of encouragement or gratitude to the lunchbox.

Coop's Creations:

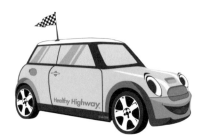

Coop and Rev eat with their eyes! They love to mix and match the foods in their meals and snacks and love to have many different bright colors: green, purple, reds, oranges, and yellows. They suggest choosing a "base" or foundation and then add ingredients to make it different every time. **This puts you in the *driver's seat* to determine the meals that you like and make your engine strong.**

PUMP IT UP:

Breakfast:
<u>Oatmeal</u> + slivered almonds + cinnamon + raisins + apples + almond butter + honey = **HIGH OCTANE FUEL!**

Lunch:
<u>Greens</u> + tomato + carrots + cucumbers + celery + beans + peppers + nuts/seeds = **HIGH CRUISING SPEED**!
Dressing: balsamic vinaigrette,

Dinner:
<u>Quinoa/rice/pasta</u> + favorite meat + sweet potato + peas + zucchini/squash = **SUPER CHARGED!**

Create your **own** specialized fuel, detailed to your own engine:
Base _____ + _____ + _____ + _____ = **FAMILY FAVORITE!**

Coop's example:
<u>Eggs</u> + spinach + avocado + tomato + quinoa patty = **SUPER CHARGED BREAKFAST!**

FUN WATER FACTS...
Do you know that water is the major component of most of your body parts?

- Our brain and heart are made up of approximately 73% water.
- Our lungs are made up of approximately 83% water.
- Our skin is made up of approximately 64% water.
- Our muscles and kidneys are made up of approximately 79% water.
- Even our bones are made up of approximately 31% water.

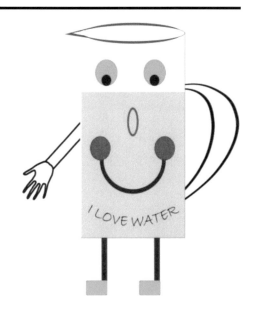

Green Light Decisions

Green-light decisions can be applied to all areas of our lives. Here are two examples of how to create a "two way" street of communication - being honest and cooperating with others.

What does it mean to be honest?

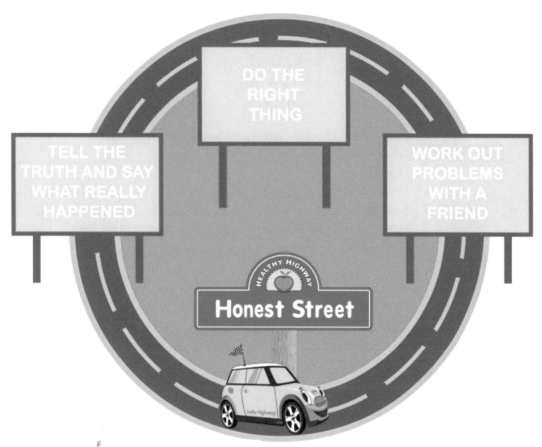

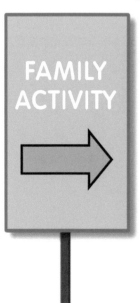

FAMILY ACTIVITY
Be truthful with your words and be willing to take responsibility for your actions...

At the end of the day discuss the following together as a family.
How does it feel when you are honest?
How does it feel when we do not tell the truth? Do you feel proud when you are honest?
How do friends respond when you tell the truth?

Red Light/Green Light Expansion
Red light/green light concept for decisions can be used in all aspects of your life, not just food choices. By applying this traffic-based model, you change red light "traffic jams" to green light "action steps." We can "re-route" and look at alternative options. Yellow light means we are being cautious, slowing down on a decision to enable us to take time to gather

information. We can move at our own speed, shift gears, and move forward to a "green light" action. This small step can lead to big changes. How exciting to start this with our children, to help them become accountable for their own healthy choices so they then become empowered to help others!

What does it mean to cooperate?

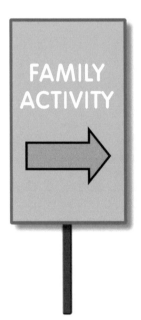

Look for opportunities during the day to...

- Say something nice to someone in your family
- Say something nice to a friend
- Help someone in your family
- Help a friend

At the end of the day discuss the following together as a family.

- How did it make you feel when you said something nice to someone?
- How did it make you feel when you did something nice for someone?
- How did it make you feel when someone did something nice for you?
- How did it make you feel when someone said something nice to you?
- How do you think the other person felt?

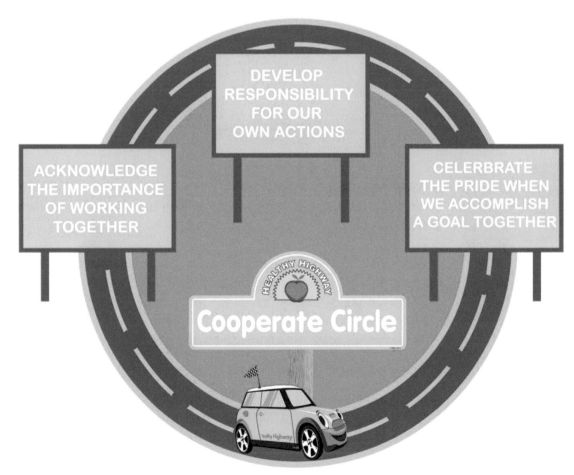

The _____ Family Road Map

Sun	Mon	Tue	Wed	Thu	Fri	Sat
30 ways for 30 healthy days.	Teach the Healthy Highway Pledge to 3 other families	Raise your awareness to all choices in the day	Encourage daily conversations of your choices with each family member.	Demonstrate your commitment to healthy choices by making 2 goals each month.	Go with the power of "green light" choices.	Be kind, be fair, be a friend.
Understand it is your innate value to be healthy.	Stop and listen to your inner GPS.	Healthy means you are in a no judgement zone.	Get in gear, any gear but park!	Keep your engine cool with lots of clean, fresh water.	Create a new green light fueled meal.	Be happy, be healthy, be strong.
Do something for yourself day.	Do not enter into stressful red light situations.	Volunteer in a local community event or business.	Celebrate your healthy choices!	Rev your engines every day with a fun activity.	Go out in the great outdoors and breathe in the fresh air!	Be honest, be positive, be grateful
	Practice your green light choices every day.	Take 10 minutes for a quiet pit stop to rejuvenate.	Do something for someone day.	Use the green light concept in all decisions you make in a day.	Laughing day.	Be proud of YOU!!
	Try a new green light food day	Take a favorite meal and make a add a healthy ingredient.	Be thankful day.	Take a favorite meal and make a add a healthy ingredient.	Smile day.	Send Rev an email about your 30 day road trip. rev@healthy-highway.com

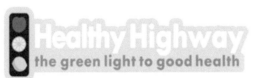

www.healthy-highway.com

The _____ Family Road Map

Sun	Mon	Tue	Wed	Thu	Fri	Sat
Healthy Highway Pledge: I promise to make MORE than one healthy choice EVERY day.	Walk for 10 minutes today.	Try a new fresh fruit.	Do sit ups during every commercial if you watch TV today.	Walk for 12 minutes.	Fuel up with a healthy breakfast.	Grocery shop and find the cereal with the lowest amount of sugar.
Have each member of your family make one part of a healthy dinner.	Walk for 15 minutes.	Do 10 push ups.	Do 10 bicep curls with a can in each hand.	Create your own salad for dinner today.	Walk for 17 minutes.	Make a healthy snack mix. Use at least 3 different types of fuels.
List 3 green light foods that you had today.	Walk for 20 minutes.	Food detective. Check your kitchen for the snack with the least sodium.	Walk up and down some stairs 10 times today!	Thirsty Thursday. Drink water all day!	Favorite Fruit Friday. Have two!	Walk for 23 minutes.
Choose 3 favorite stretches. Try to add 5 more reps to each one.	Walk for 24 minutes.	Draw a picture of your family exercising and put it on the fridge!	Wellness Wednesday. Choose a favorite activity and have fun!	Choose 2 veggies for your snack today.	Fitness Friday Do 3 sets of 10 "green bean leans" (wall push ups).	Walk for 25 minutes.
List all the foods you eat today on a traffic light poster!	Dance to your favorite music for 2 minutes.	Can you walk 30 minutes today?	Celebrate your healthy choices.	List 2 goals.	Name 2 new foods that you tried that you liked. Name your favorite activity.	Did you meet your goals? Talk about what you liked during this month.

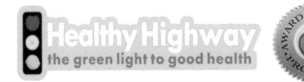

www.healthy-highway.com

The _____ Family Road Map

Sun	Mon	Tue	Wed	Thu	Fri	Sat
Make a list of activities to "rev" your engine for each day of the week.	Talk about each nutrition rule on your placemat at dinner and why you think they are important.	Choose 2 new goals for the month.	Create a new game for the family to play with items you find in your home.	Walk for 20 minutes.	List 2 new veggies to try for next week.	Find a park and explore. Take a healthy snack and water.
Start a garden. Use pots indoors or plant outside.	Choose a number of healthy choices for the week and use your fuel gauge.	Go outside and play catch as a family.	Talk about the 2 new veggies and what you liked or didn't like about them.	Write an email to Rev and tell him your favorite healthy choice of the week.	Make a healthy breakfast together to start your engines.	Make a healthy trail mix snack and ask your friends over to try it.
Go for a power walk after dinner.	Decide what each member of the family will make for Wednesday night dinner.	Try a new sport.	Play traffic bingo in the car - Try to find all 6 nutrition traffic signs.	Go on an alphabet hunt. Find something that starts with each letter of the alphabet.	Discover a new area to hike through.	Choose 2 new fruits to try.
Ask friends or family over and prepare a "green light" meal for them.	Have a picnic... inside or outside. Fill the basket with green light foods.	Go for a bike ride.	Design a car out of cardboard and "drive" it across the yard. Have a race!	Find a playground and go on all the equipment.	Make a "veggie vehicle" out of vegetables. Email a picture of it to Coop!	Have friends over and make an obstacle course in the backyard.
Take a "healthy-selfie: picture of your family exercising. Email it to Wendy.	Be proud of your "engine and make a special "healthy fuel" dinner!					

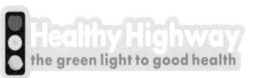

www.healthy-highway.com

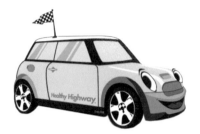

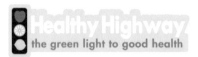
Healthy Highway
the green light to good health

Rev your Engines

How to Get Started:

1. Set a family goal or "destination" by describing a change you would like to make to increase healthy decisions.

2. Write that goal down and post where everyone can see it.

3. Choose a time frame to complete the goal: i.e. 1 week; 2 weeks; 1 month

4. Write down action steps to reach your goal.

5. Use the "Family Road Map" calendars on the previous pages to help you start down the road to healthy choices.

6. As a family, decide how you want to celebrate "crossing the finish line"of meeting your goal.

   Set a new goal!

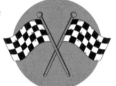

Want to make healthy choices easy for your family?
Invite them to be creative and use these amazing visuals every day!

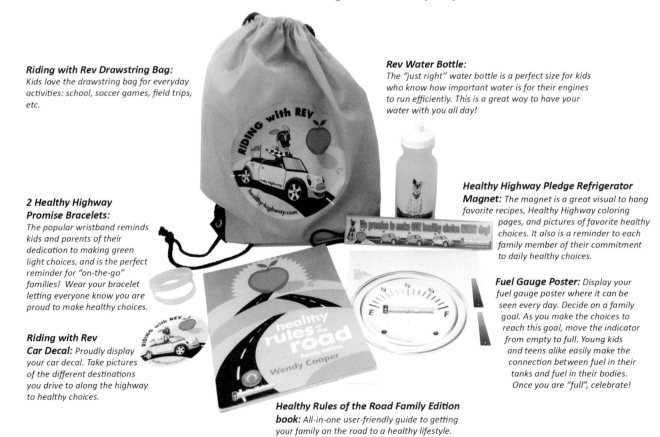

Riding with Rev Drawstring Bag:
Kids love the drawstring bag for everyday activities: school, soccer games, field trips, etc.

2 Healthy Highway Promise Bracelets:
The popular wristband reminds kids and parents of their dedication to making green light choices, and is the perfect reminder for "on-the-go" families! Wear your bracelet letting everyone know you are proud to make healthy choices.

Riding with Rev Car Decal: *Proudly display your car decal. Take pictures of the different destinations you drive to along the highway to healthy choices.*

Rev Water Bottle:
The "just right" water bottle is a perfect size for kids who know how important water is for their engines to run efficiently. This is a great way to have your water with you all day!

Healthy Highway Pledge Refrigerator Magnet: *The magnet is a great visual to hang favorite recipes, Healthy Highway coloring pages, and pictures of favorite healthy choices. It also is a reminder to each family member of their commitment to daily healthy choices.*

Fuel Gauge Poster: *Display your fuel gauge poster where it can be seen every day. Decide on a family goal. As you make the choices to reach this goal, move the indicator from empty to full. Young kids and teens alike easily make the connection between fuel in their tanks and fuel in their bodies. Once you are "full", celebrate!*

Healthy Rules of the Road Family Edition book: *All-in-one user-friendly guide to getting your family on the road to a healthy lifestyle.*

Visit the website to order your own Riding with Rev Pack! www.healthy-highway.com

Healthy Highway - *Rules of the Road* License Plate Award

CONGRATULATIONS!

After you have completed your monthly goals, place your family photo on the "State of Good Health" License Plate award (below) and proudly display for families and friends to see.

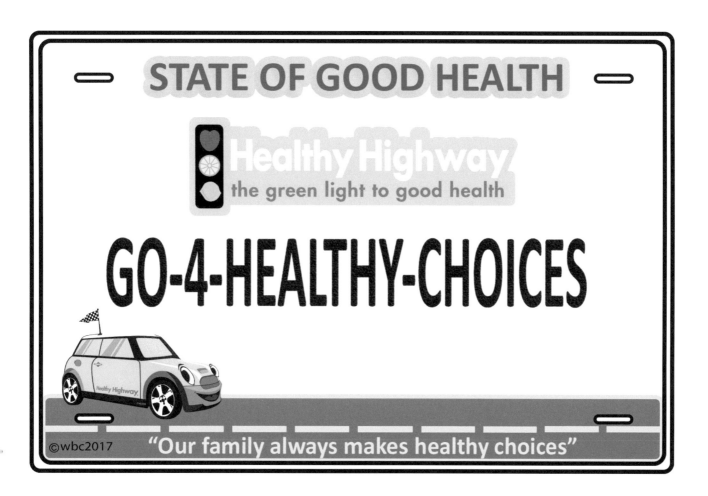

Road to Success

Never-ending road trip for a happy and strong engine.......

We have one *engine*.....we have the opportunity to have a *top performance engine* that will run smoothly and efficiently our entire lives. But we need to take time to take care of it, giving it the best fuels we can, maintaining it with tune-ups, providing it with plenty of water, and keeping it strong with exercise and activity. Choices are made each day that will lead us on the highway to health. Be proud of those choices, understand the strength of those choices, and enjoy the journey. Understand that when challenges occur, it is our engine letting us know we need to stop, recalculate, and be aware of the decisions that have caused this bump in the road of not feeling well in some manner.

I am grateful to be able to share this lifestyle journey with you. It is my gift to you. Here is your owner's guarantee. Please continue to take responsibility for this magnificent engine:

- You are the sole owner, therefore having complete power to make choices designed specifically for your body and health.
  Think about the choices you make, be aware, and modify as needed.
- Follow your inner GPS. It knows exactly what is needed for your body to be strong and healthy.
- Expect results: feeling good, feeling strong, having energy, being positive, and being proud.

Always believe in the power of healthy foods and green-light decisions.

Wendy

BE A DRIVING FORCE. JOIN THE HEALTHY REV-OLUTION!

Share your healthy choices with other friends and families. Invite them to join you on the Healthy Highway. Take the Healthy Highway Pledge: "We promise to make at least one healthy choice every day." Once you take the pledge, email me saying you would like to join the "Rev-olution" and I will send you a Revolution Award certificate. wcooper@healthy-highway.com

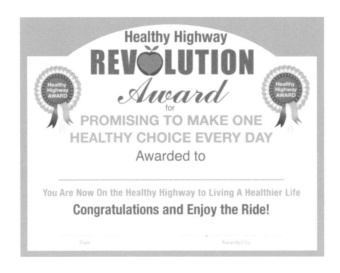

My Story

It has been quite a road trip! About fifteen years ago physical education teachers like myself were given the charge of incorporating nutrition into their curriculum. How can I keep the children moving and having fun while teaching them about healthy lifestyles? I decided to use traffic metaphors to teach my students to "drive" safely and take care of their "engines". As they say, the rest is history.

As I watched my students embrace this theme, I knew I wanted to share it with other professionals and families. I had the opportunity to travel the country presenting at state and national health and physical education conferences. I was able to work with school districts and watch my program grow and include new ideas I never had thought of. Then I published a book, Healthy Rules of the Road Family Edition, which has fun tools to add to the excitement of the program.

I would like my readers to understand that they have one "engine" and that it can run at top performance all the time. But we need to take time and take care of it, giving it the best fuels, maintaining it with "tune ups", providing it with plenty of water, and keeping it strong with exercise and activity. Be proud of the choices being made and understand challenges will occur. All we need to do is recalculate and move forward. Follow and listen to your inner GPS since your body knows what it needs. Always believe in the power of green light decisions

As parents, we have the unique opportunity to fuel the future by helping our children adopt healthy lifestyles. We can serve as what I like to call role models or "road models" by applying the Healthy Highway Rules of the Road.

All of this came from my heart, and it was only recently that I noticed the real reason for the heart in the apple of my Healthy Highway cover. When it was designed, I felt the apple was for nutrition and the heart was for activity. That was correct at that time, but over the course of these 15 years, it now represents MY heart. I love how Healthy Highway has evolved into the family edition – it is an invitation for you to join me on the road to healthy choices, as the main driver in determining the best healthy lifestyle choices to meet your own family's individual needs.

This is a trip of a lifetime …
welcome to the state of good health!

From my heart to yours,

Wendy H Cooper

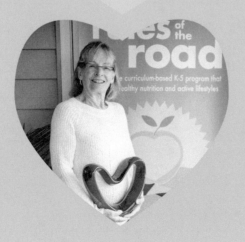

Rev's Activity Kit for Kids

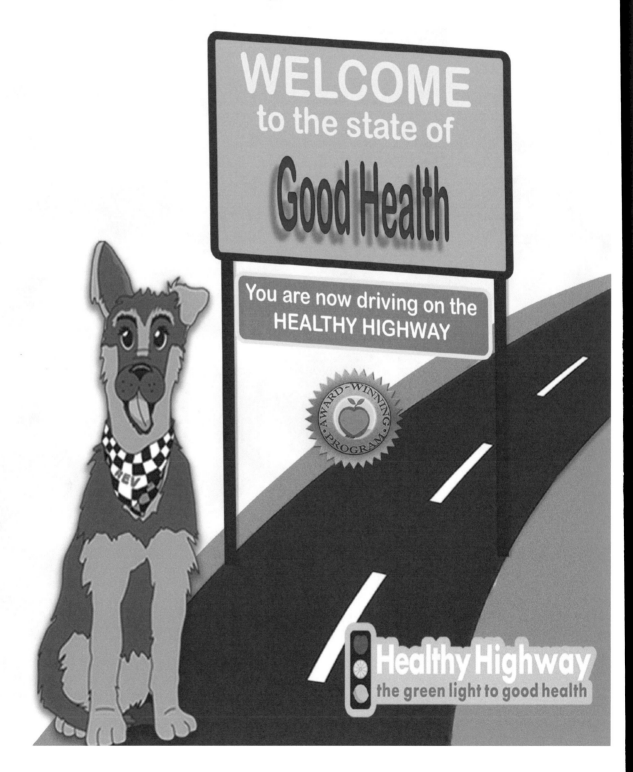

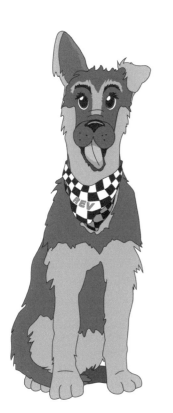

Welcome to the Healthy Highway! I am Rev, the Healthy Highway mascot who will help guide you to healthy choices. The theme of this program is to think of your body as a car engine that needs healthy foods or "fuels" to make it strong. I learned about being healthy from my best friend Wendy Cooper.

Thanks for traveling down the road to healthy choices with me. Have fun with the activity pages that you can copy and display in your home. It will be an exciting ride!

Rev

healthy
rules of the
road

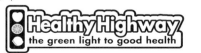

©wbc 2016

Healthy Highway Pledge:

I have been lucky to watch families choose healthy choices every day. I met one family that had so much fun working together and helping each other make healthy choices that I wrote this Healthy Highway Pledge. Say this with your family everyday:

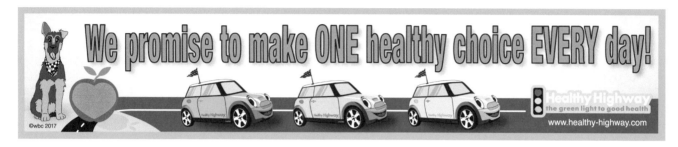

Healthy Highway "Rev-olution":

Be a driving force and join the Healthy Highway Revolution! Help others to make healthy choices. It helps to connect with other kids on this highway and it is a lot more fun with more people.

Wendy and I want lots of drivers on the Healthy Highway so we need your help. Find three friends or families that might like your healthy "knowledge" and share what you have learned while being on the Healthy Highway. Email how you helped others to make healthy choices to: Rev@healthy-highway.com

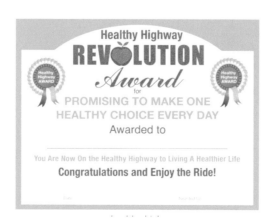

Can you find the hidden Rules of the Road words below?

Rev
Coop
Cruise
Engine
Fuel
Fun
Green light
Healthy
Highway
Road map

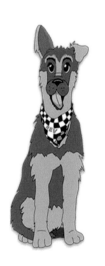

T	J	C	A	R	L	H	Y	T	O
R	H	K	H	I	G	H	W	A	Y
O	M	G	I	E	T	T	N	V	H
A	R	E	I	N	I	G	N	E	T
D	S	P	S	L	L	C	U	R	L
M	N	I	I	E	N	E	F	H	A
A	K	S	U	W	Z	E	U	O	E
P	B	F	R	R	T	L	E	A	H
R	E	Q	C	C	O	O	P	R	A
R	E	P	V	G	H	W	A	Y	G

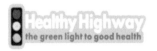

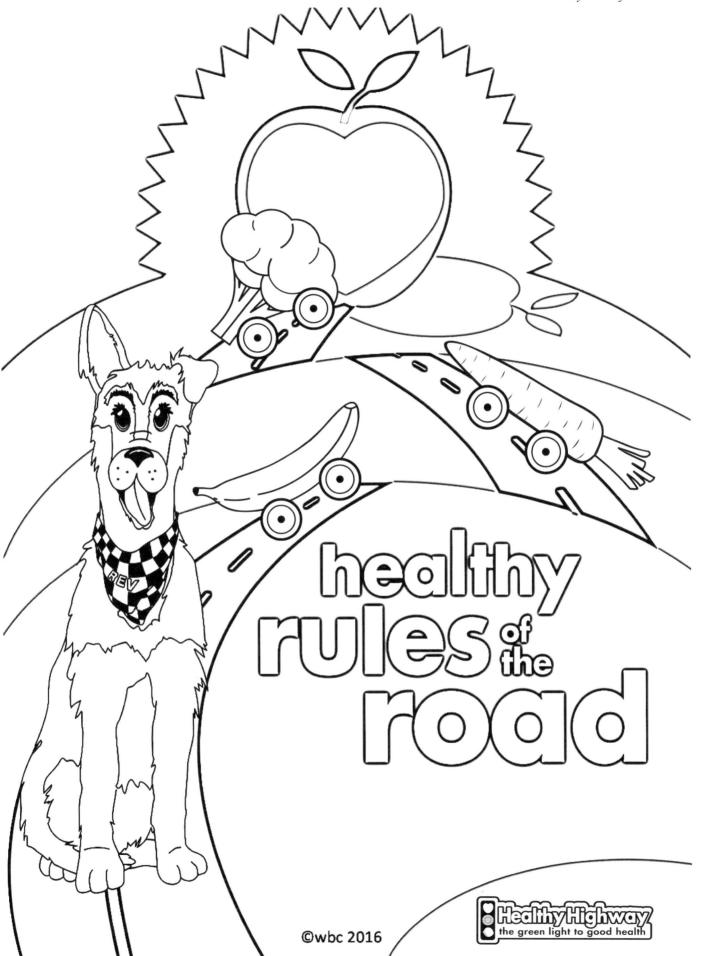

©wbc 2016

©wbc2017

Nutrition

RULE #1
- Stop for
- Healthy
- Snacks

RULE #2
- To
- Five
- A day

RULE #3
- Watch for oils
- Slow down on fats
- Pass by sugar

RULE #4
- Always
- Eat
- Breakfast

RULE #5
- Junk food
- Soda
- Candy

RULE #6
- Be happy
- Be healthy
- Be strong

Rev's Advice

www.Healthy-Highway.com

"Fill your tank" with high performance fuels

"Rev" your engine everyday with plenty of exercise

"Fill up" with water several times a day

Healthy Highway
the green light to good health

Safety

RULE #1
- Go
- For
- Healthy Choices

RULE #2
- Keep hot foods hot
- Keep cold foods cold
- Store all foods

RULE #3
- Watch for hot surfaces
- Respect kitchen tools
- Clean all surfaces

RULE #4
- Always
- Wash
- Hands

RULE #5
- Without
- Adult
- Supervision

RULE #6
- Be safe
- Be creative
- Have fun

Welcome to Rev's Vegetable Garden!

Rev has some delicious and very healthy vegetables growing in his garden this year. You'll find the list below. Can you find them in the word search to the right?

Asparagus
Avocado
Broccoli
Carrots
Cauliflower
Cucumber
Eggplant
Endive
Garden Salad
Green Beans
Jicama
Kale
Lima Beans
Lentils
Navy Beans
Peas
Peppers
Spinach
Raw Veggies
Vegetable Soup
Yams
Yellow Peppers
Zucchini

```
C G W O X B A N P Q S C L H Z F D L A M Z V J A M R
F D L D M C Y E L L O W P E P P E R S C L S G I E M
A T V A G A R A S A L A E B E A S H A O S V X J K A
V E G C A B K L E R O C A K A L S G A R D N P E A K
K M L O A S P A R A G U S Z S C C H I S M A X J A E
M D I V E G G P L A R N T S O U P V E G G I K K R H
T S M A C A U L I E E B A E S N G E G G P L A N T E
Y Z F C R N J L B C E S I A D M O N S Q J M H R L A
D Q S N A V Y B E A N S I V E N W D V Z A M K S A L
F K D K X K O L L J B R O C C O L I H C V M S Q R T
E J N T R W L Y K C E U O N R O C V I P I N A C C H
J I K H E K E L E J A B E N N S J J L E M A B E A Y
V M I O W A S P A I N I H C C U Z R A G U S W E O C
E A G V O S O P E Q S R W V E G H G I E S S H O P H
G M D A L A S N E D R A G N Q X A B E A S A L E K O
E L M K F K K A C U C U M B E R L E T U C E B R S I
T B A J I C K S T R O S N A E B A M I L S A P E L C
A E A C L H E P E P E R S I W Z I L U C I C C E
B A P U U K U P E K J I A M A C S B E T T G H E R S
L F P C A L E E S P O E A S A C L N L I G I M A B E
E Y H U C E K L E B P C A R P R T O T E L R U W L B
S A E Y A S P A R A G E A P E I K O V P K S T V Q L
O X P O I H R Y B Q R R R S L L N W J I S S A P P Q
U T P L D O E B B Q A L P S W E A A A P O W P I W L
P G E T R M V G R E E N M A X R U W C A V A N I M A
L I R E M E A R E D C A R R O T S K Y H Y O U G A Q
X Y S A N S T K S A Y P O G S L A D B E E N S C C M
```

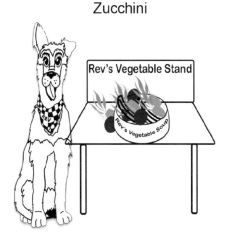

Rev's Vegetable Stand

Rev's Vegetable Soup

Can you find Rev's Hidden Message?
Hint: It is something we are doing when we eat nutritious foods.

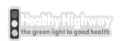
the green light to good health

Something to share with your family & friends....

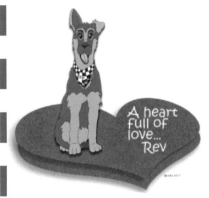

FREE COUPON FROM...REV

A little present from me to you...
There is something that I hope you will do...
Exercise and be really smart...
My gift to you is a walk for your heart.

No expiration/Reusable/Grows as you give to more people

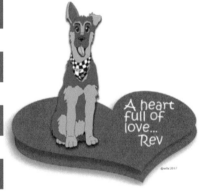

FREE COUPON FROM...REV

A little present from me to you...
There is something that I hope you will do...
Exercise and be really smart...
My gift to you is a walk for your heart.

No expiration/Reusable/Grows as you give to more people

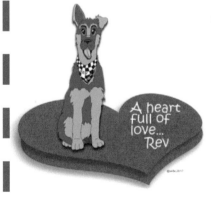

FREE COUPON FROM...REV

A little present from me to you...
There is something that I hope you will do...
Exercise and be really smart...
My gift to you is a walk for your heart.

No expiration/Reusable/Grows as you give to more people

Become a Chef on the Healthy Highway...

Create your own healthy recipes using the Healthy Highway Recipe Card provided below. Create as many healthy recipes as you like using green light ingredients.

Copy and share them with your family and friends...

"I can't be up front with the adults in a car and be a driver...but I can be the driver in the kitchen." - Sophia V. 9 years old

Recipe for: _____

From _____ Kitchen...

Ingredients...   Directions...

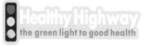

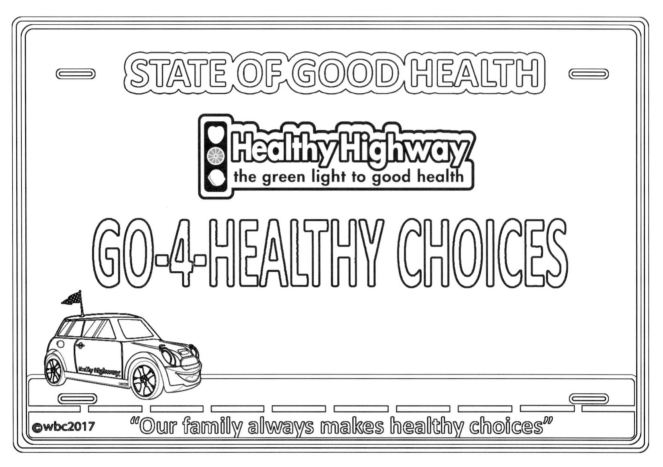

How can you get your ideas and stories to me?

I can't get to all of your homes but you can send your ideas to me. Ask your parents to email your letters and messages to me at rev@healthy-highway.com. Be sure to let me know that I can share your messages with all of your friends driving on the Healthy Highway since it is like belonging to a club, a healthy club. Tell your friends they can write to me too. All your great ideas will make Healthy Highway bigger and better!

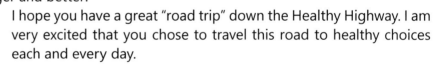

I hope you have a great "road trip" down the Healthy Highway. I am very excited that you chose to travel this road to healthy choices each and every day.

Be happy, healthy, strong and kind.

With love from my heart to yours,

Rev

Answer key for Hidden Words...

```
T  J  C  A  R  L  H  Y  T  O
R  H  K  H  I  G  H  W  A  Y
O  M  G  I  E  T  T  N  V  H
A  R  E  I  N  I  G  N  E  T
D  S  P  S  L  L  C  U  R  L
M  N  I  E  N  E  F  H  A
A  K  S  U  W  Z  E  U  O  E
P  B  F  R  R  T  L  E  A  H
R  E  Q  C  C  O  O  P  R  A
R  E  P  V  G  H  W  A  Y  G
```

```
C  G  W O X  B  A  N  P  Q  S  C  L  H  Z  F  D  L  A  M  Z  V  J  A  M  R
F  D  L  D  M  C  Y  E  L  L  O  W  P  E  P  P  E  R  S  C  L  S  G  I  E  M
A  T  V  A  G  A  R  A  S  A  L  A  E  B  E  A  S  H  A  O  S  V  X  J  K  A
V  E  G  C  A  B  K  L  E  R  O  C  A  K  A  L  S  G  A  R  D  N  P  E  A  K
K  M  L  O  A  S  P  A  R  A  G  U  S  Z  U  C  C  H  I  S  M  A  X  J  A  E
M  D  I  V  E  G  G  P  L  A  R  N  T  S  O  U  P  V  E  G  G  I  K  K  R  H
T  S  M  A  C  A  U  L  I  E  E  B  A  E  S  N  G  E  G  G  P  L  A  N  T  E
Y  Z  F  C  R  N  J  L  B  C  E  S  I  A  D  M  O  N  S  Q  J  C  H  R  L  A
D  Q  S  N  A  V  Y  B  E  A  N  S  I  V  E  N  W  D  V  Z  I  M  K  S  A  L
F  K  D  K  X  K  O  L  L  J  B  R  O  C  C  O  L  I  H  J  V  M  S  Q  R  T
E  J  N  T  R  W  L  Y  K  C  E  U  O  N  R  O  C  V  A  P  I  N  A  C  C  H
J  I  K  H  E  K  E  L  E  J  A  B  E  N  N  S  J  E  L  E  M  A  B  E  A  Y
V  M  I  O  W  A  S  P  A  I  N  I  H  C  C  U  Z  R  A  G  U  S  W  E  O  C
E  A  G  V  O  S  O  P  E  Q  S  R  W  V  E  G  H  G  I  E  S  S  H  O  P  H
G  M  D  A  L  A  S  N  E  D  R  A  G  N  Q  X  A  B  E  A  S  A  L  E  K  O
E  L  M     F  K  K  A  C  U  C  U  M  B  E  R  L  E  T  U  C  E  B  R  E  I
T  B  A  J  I  C  K  S  T  R  O  S  N  A  E  B  A  M  I  L  S  A  P  I  L  C
A  E  A  C  L  H  E  P  E  P  E  R  S  I  W  Z  I  L  U  C  G  C  C  E
B  A  P  U  U  K  U  P  E  K  J  I  A  M  A  C  S  B  E  T  T  G  H  E  R  S
L  F  P  C  A  L  E  E  S  P  O  E  A  S  A  C  L  N  L  I  E  I  M  A  B  E
E  Y  H  U  C  E  K  L  E  B  P  C  A  R  P  R  T  O  T  V  L  R  U  W  L  B
S  A  E  Y  A  S  P  A  R  A  G  E  A  P  E  I  K  O  W  P  K  S  T  V  Q  L
O  X  P  O  I  H  R  Y  B  Q  R  R  R  S  L  L  N  A  J  I  S  S  A  P  P  Q
U  T  P  L  D  O  E  B  B  Q  A  L  P  S  W  E  R  A  A  P  O  W  P  I  W  L
P  G  E  T  R  M  V  G  R  E  E  N  M  A  X  M  U  W  C  A  V  A  N  I  M  A
L  I  R  E  M  E  A  R  E  D  C  A  R  R  O  T  S  K  Y  H  Y  O  U  G  A  Q
X  Y  S  A  N  S  T  K  S  A  Y  P  O  G  S  L  A  D  B  E  E  N  S  C  C  M
```

Hidden Message Answer: Make Healthy Choices

Printed in the United States
By Bookmasters